Effective Natural Healing and Prevention of Seborrheic Dermatitis

The Complete Step-by-Step Practical Guide to Clear, Radiant, Healthy Skin and Lasting Relief

Nelson Andrew

BONUS: Simple, effective DIY recipes to nourish your skin and support natural healing.

Table of Contents

Chapter 1: Understanding Seborrheic Dermatitis
1.1 What is Seborrheic Dermatitis?
1.2 Symptoms and Triggers
1.3 The Role of Skin Health in Seborrheic Dermatitis

Chapter 2: The Holistic Approach to Healing
2.1 Why Conventional Treatments Fall Short
2.2 The Power of Holistic Healing
2.3 Integrating Body, Mind, and Skin Health

Chapter 3: Diet and Nutrition for Healthy Skin
3.1 Anti-Inflammatory Foods
3.2 Gut Health and Skin Connection
3.3 Foods to Avoid for Flare Prevention

Chapter 4: Natural Remedies and Topical Solutions
4.1 Essential Oils and Herbal Treatments
4.2 DIY Natural Skincare Recipes
4.3 Safe and Effective Over-the-Counter Options

Chapter 5: Stress Management and Emotional Well-Being
5.1 The Stress-Skin Connection
5.2 Mindfulness, Meditation, and Relaxation Techniques
5.3 Creating a Balanced Lifestyle for Skin Health

Chapter 6: Detoxifying Your Environment
6.1 Identifying Harmful Chemicals and Irritants
6.2 Switching to Natural Skincare and Household Products
6.3 Creating a Skin-Healthy Living Space

Chapter 7: Building a Flare-Free Skincare Routine
7.1 Daily Skincare Practices for Seborrheic Dermatitis

7.2 How to Properly Cleanse, Moisturize, and Protect

7.3 Adjusting Your Routine During Flare-Ups

Chapter 8: Healing From Within: Supplements and Nutritional Support

8.1 Key Vitamins and Minerals for Skin Health

8.2 Probiotics and Gut Support

8.3 The Role of Omega-3s and Antioxidants

Chapter 9: Preventing Future Flare-Ups

Chapter 1

Understanding Seborrheic Dermatitis

1.1 What is Seborrheic Dermatitis?

Seborrheic dermatitis is a common, chronic skin condition that causes red, inflamed, and scaly patches, often accompanied by itching and flaking. It primarily affects areas of the skin rich in oil glands, such as the scalp, face, chest, and upper back. When it occurs on the scalp, it is often referred to as dandruff or cradle cap in infants.

1.2 Symptoms and Triggers

1. Flaky Skin: Yellowish or white scales, often greasy, on the scalp, face, or other affected areas.

2. Red Patches: Inflamed, red, or pink areas of skin.

3. Itchiness: Mild to intense itching, sometimes accompanied by a burning sensation.

4. Greasy Appearance: Skin may appear shiny or oily in affected areas.

5. Crusting: In severe cases, crusty plaques can form.

6. Dandruff: Persistent flaking of the scalp, often confused with regular dandruff.

7. Affected Areas: Commonly includes the scalp, eyebrows, eyelids, sides of the nose, ears, chest, and upper back.

8. Worsening in Cold Weather: Symptoms tend to be more severe in winter or dry conditions.

Common Triggers

1. Stress: Emotional or physical stress can exacerbate symptoms.

2. Weather Changes: Cold, dry winters or hot, humid climates can worsen the condition.

3. Hormonal Fluctuations: Changes in hormone levels, such as during puberty, pregnancy, or menopause.

4. Certain Medications: Psychotropic drugs and some immune-suppressing medications may aggravate symptoms.

5. Yeast Overgrowth: Overgrowth of Malassezia yeast on the skin can trigger or worsen inflammation.

6. Skin Irritants: Harsh soaps, detergents, or alcohol-based skin products.

7. Dietary Factors: High-sugar, high-fat, or low-nutrient diets can sometimes contribute.

8. Lack of Proper Hygiene: Excess oil build-up due to infrequent washing.

9. Genetic Factors: Family history of similar conditions or skin sensitivities.

10. Underlying Conditions: Conditions like Parkinson's disease, HIV, or other immune-related issues can increase the risk.

1.3 The Role of Skin Health in Seborrheic Dermatitis

While Seborrheic dermatitis exact cause is multifactorial—ranging from genetic predisposition to environmental triggers—skin health plays a pivotal role in both the development and management of the condition.

1. Skin Barrier Function

The skin barrier is the body's first line of defense, protecting against irritants, allergens, and pathogens. In seborrheic dermatitis, this barrier is often compromised, allowing external irritants to penetrate and exacerbate inflammation. Weak or damaged skin barriers can lead to dryness and sensitivity, making skin more vulnerable to the overgrowth of Malassezia yeast, a key factor associated with seborrheic dermatitis.

Strengthening the skin barrier through proper hydration, gentle cleansers, and moisturizers enriched with ceramides or fatty acids is essential. These measures help restore the skin's natural defense, reducing inflammation and flakiness.

2. Oil Production and Balance

Seborrheic dermatitis often occurs in areas with high sebaceous (oil-producing) gland activity. Excess oil can create an environment where Malassezia thrives, leading to irritation and scaling. However, overly dry skin can also exacerbate symptoms, as the skin compensates by producing more oil. Maintaining balanced oil production is critical.

This can be achieved by avoiding harsh cleansers that strip natural oils and incorporating skin-friendly oils like jojoba or squalane to maintain equilibrium.

3. Microbiome Health

A healthy skin microbiome is essential for preventing skin disorders. The microbiome consists of various microorganisms that coexist on the skin's surface, maintaining its health and resilience. In seborrheic dermatitis, an imbalance in the microbiome—particularly the overgrowth of Malassezia—can trigger symptoms.

Promoting microbiome health through prebiotic and probiotic skincare can help maintain balance. Ingredients such as oat extract or fermented products support the skin's natural microbial diversity, reducing the likelihood of flare-ups.

4. Inflammation Control

Chronic inflammation underlies seborrheic dermatitis, contributing to redness, itching, and discomfort. Managing inflammation requires a multi-faceted approach, **including:**

Using anti-inflammatory ingredients like aloe vera, calendula, or chamomile in skincare.

Avoiding known irritants, such as harsh soaps, fragrances, or alcohol-based products.

Supporting the skin's repair mechanisms with antioxidants like vitamin E or green tea extract.

5. Lifestyle and Nutrition

Healthy skin starts from within. Diet, hydration, and stress management play a significant role in maintaining skin health and controlling seborrheic dermatitis. A diet rich in omega-3 fatty acids, antioxidants, and vitamins A, C, and E supports skin repair and reduces inflammation.

Staying hydrated keeps the skin supple, while managing stress—through practices like mindfulness or yoga—helps regulate hormonal fluctuations that may influence sebaceous gland activity.

6. Personalized Skincare Routine

Building a skincare routine tailored to individual skin needs is vital. **Key elements include:**

Cleansing: Use gentle, sulfate-free cleansers to remove dirt without stripping moisture.

Exfoliation: Mild exfoliation with ingredients like salicylic acid or lactic acid can reduce flaking without irritating sensitive skin.

Moisturizing: Opt for non-comedogenic, hypoallergenic moisturizers to maintain hydration.

Skin health is central to understanding and managing seborrheic dermatitis. By focusing on strengthening the skin barrier, balancing oil production, supporting microbiome diversity, controlling inflammation, and adopting a skin-friendly lifestyle, individuals can reduce symptoms and improve their quality of life. Consistent, thoughtful care of the skin ensures long-term management of this condition and fosters overall skin wellness.

Chapter 2

<u>The Holistic Approach to Healing</u>

2.1 Why Conventional Treatments Fall Short

Conventional treatments, while widely used, frequently fall short of providing lasting relief. Understanding why this happens sheds light on the importance of a holistic approach to healing.

The Limitations of Conventional Treatments

1. Symptom Management Over Root Causes

Most conventional treatments focus on alleviating symptoms rather than addressing the underlying causes. Corticosteroids, antifungal creams, and medicated shampoos may temporarily reduce redness or scaling but do little to prevent recurrence. This approach often traps individuals in a cycle of flare-ups and dependency on treatments.

2. Potential Side Effects

Long-term use of certain medications can lead to adverse effects. For example, corticosteroids may thin the skin or cause rebound flares when discontinued. Similarly, antifungal treatments can disrupt the natural skin microbiome, potentially worsening the problem over time.

3. Overlooking Individual Variations

Conventional treatments are often designed for broad application, ignoring individual differences in lifestyle, diet, stress levels, or genetic predispositions. What works for one person may fail entirely for another, leaving many without a tailored solution.

4. Temporary Solutions

Conventional methods frequently address the external manifestations of seborrheic dermatitis without considering internal contributors like inflammation, hormonal imbalances, or gut health. As a result, treatments can provide relief only as long as they are used, offering no long-term resolution.

The Holistic Approach: A Path to Lasting Healing

Holistic healing shifts the focus from suppressing symptoms to restoring overall health and balance. It considers the body as an interconnected system, emphasizing prevention and sustainable wellness.

1. Addressing Internal Imbalances

Seborrheic dermatitis often reflects internal issues such as inflammation, poor gut health, or stress. A holistic approach involves identifying and correcting these imbalances through diet, hydration, and targeted supplementation. Foods rich in omega-3 fatty acids, probiotics, and anti-inflammatory nutrients can support skin health from within.

2. Nurturing the Skin's Natural Barrier

The skin's barrier is essential for protecting against irritants and maintaining hydration. Gentle, natural skincare products free of harsh chemicals can help rebuild and maintain this barrier, reducing flare-ups over time.

3. Stress Management

Chronic stress exacerbates seborrheic dermatitis by disrupting hormonal balance and weakening the immune system. Holistic healing emphasizes practices like meditation, yoga, and adequate sleep to lower stress levels and improve skin health.

4. Balancing the Microbiome

The skin and gut microbiomes play a crucial role in managing seborrheic dermatitis. Probiotic-rich foods, prebiotics, and avoiding overly harsh cleansers can help restore this balance, reducing the likelihood of inflammation and irritation.

5. Customized Care

A holistic approach recognizes that everyone's triggers and needs are unique. Through careful observation and lifestyle adjustments, individuals can identify factors—such as specific foods, environmental conditions, or stressors—that worsen their condition.

Prevention Through Holistic Practices

Prevention is a cornerstone of holistic healing. Regular self-care practices, such as maintaining a nutrient-rich diet, staying hydrated, and protecting the skin from extreme weather conditions, can significantly reduce the risk of flare-ups. Routine mindfulness practices and balancing work-life demands can further support overall well-being.

Why Holistic Healing Works

Unlike conventional treatments, a holistic approach empowers individuals to take charge of their health. By addressing the root causes of seborrheic dermatitis and promoting long-term balance, this method provides lasting relief and often eliminates the need for dependency on medications. While it requires patience and commitment, the rewards—a healthier body, clearer skin, and improved quality of life—are well worth the effort.

In embracing a holistic path, individuals transform not only their skin but also their overall health, achieving harmony that conventional treatments often fail to deliver.

2.2 The Power of Holistic Healing

While modern medicine offers a variety of treatments, from medicated shampoos to topical creams, these approaches often focus on managing symptoms rather than addressing the root cause. This is where the holistic approach to healing comes into play — a comprehensive, all-encompassing method that looks at the body as a whole and aims to restore balance from within.

What is a Holistic Approach to Healing?

Holistic healing is a philosophy that emphasizes the interconnectedness of the mind, body, and spirit. Rather than isolating a specific illness or part of the body, holistic practitioners look at how different aspects of a person's life impact their overall well-being. This approach recognizes that physical symptoms are often linked to emotional, mental, and even spiritual factors. In the case of seborrheic dermatitis, holistic healing seeks to address not just the skin condition itself, but to explore the underlying imbalances that may be contributing to it.

Key Principles of Holistic Healing

1. Treating the Whole Person: Holistic healing considers all aspects of a person's health — physical, mental, emotional, and spiritual. It does not treat seborrheic dermatitis as a standalone issue but as a symptom of a larger imbalance in the body.

2. Prevention First: Rather than focusing solely on treating symptoms, holistic healing emphasizes prevention. This might involve lifestyle changes, dietary adjustments, stress management, and other practices that support the body's natural ability to heal and maintain balance.

3. Natural Healing Methods: Holistic healing often relies on natural remedies and therapies, such as herbal treatments, nutritional adjustments, acupuncture, and mindfulness practices, rather than harsh medications that can have side effects.

4. Self-Care and Empowerment: A holistic approach encourages individuals to take an active role in their healing process. Patients are empowered to make informed choices about their health, often learning new ways to care for their bodies and prevent future flare-ups.

Understanding Seborrheic Dermatitis Holistically

Possible Causes

Seborrheic dermatitis is often linked to an overgrowth of yeast on the skin, but there are many contributing factors that can trigger or worsen the condition. **From a holistic perspective, the following factors are considered:**

Diet and Nutrition: Poor nutrition or food sensitivities can exacerbate inflammation in the body, making skin conditions like seborrheic dermatitis worse. A diet high in processed foods, sugars, and unhealthy fats may contribute to flare-ups.

Stress and Emotional Health: Stress is known to weaken the immune system, making the body more susceptible to various conditions, including skin disorders. Emotional imbalances, such as anxiety or unresolved trauma, can manifest physically on the skin.

Gut Health: The connection between gut health and skin health is well-established. Imbalances in gut bacteria, inflammation, or poor digestion can contribute to skin issues like seborrheic dermatitis.

Environmental Factors: External factors such as weather, pollution, or exposure to harsh chemicals can irritate the skin. Holistic healing takes these into account and seeks to minimize exposure to harmful environmental triggers.

Holistic Approaches to Treat and Prevent Seborrheic Dermatitis

1. Dietary Adjustments:

A nutrient-dense, anti-inflammatory diet can help reduce seborrheic dermatitis symptoms. Some holistic practitioners recommend eliminating common allergens like dairy, gluten, and sugar, which can trigger inflammation. Consuming foods rich in omega-3 fatty acids (found in fish and flaxseed) can also help reduce inflammation. Fermented foods like yogurt or kimchi can promote a healthy gut, which is crucial for skin health.

2. Stress Management:

Since stress can exacerbate seborrheic dermatitis, managing stress is a key component of holistic healing. This may involve practices such as meditation, yoga, breathing exercises, or spending time in nature. These activities help calm the nervous system, reduce inflammation, and support overall well-being.

3. Natural Topical Treatments:
Instead of using medicated creams, which can sometimes cause side effects, holistic healing often recommends natural remedies. For instance, coconut oil and tea tree oil have antifungal properties that may help reduce yeast overgrowth on the skin. Aloe vera and chamomile can soothe inflamed skin, providing relief from itching and redness.

4. Probiotics and Digestive Health:
Supporting gut health is essential for many skin conditions, including seborrheic dermatitis. Probiotics, either through supplements or fermented foods, can help balance the gut

microbiome, which in turn helps regulate inflammation and improve skin health.

5. Herbal Remedies:
Herbs like burdock root, dandelion, and turmeric are known for their anti-inflammatory and detoxifying properties. These can be consumed as teas or supplements to help cleanse the body and reduce inflammation, ultimately benefiting the skin.

6. Acupuncture and Traditional Chinese Medicine (TCM):
Acupuncture is often used in holistic treatment to balance the body's energy (Qi) and improve circulation. In TCM, seborrheic dermatitis may be viewed as an imbalance in the body's internal heat or dampness, and acupuncture or specific herbal formulas may be prescribed to address these imbalances.

7. Maintaining a Healthy Scalp and Skin Care Routine:

Using natural, gentle products on the scalp and skin can help prevent irritation. Avoiding harsh shampoos, soaps, and chemicals can reduce the risk of triggering flare-ups. Regularly washing with mild, natural cleansers, and moisturizing with plant-based oils can help keep the skin calm and hydrated.

The Benefits of a Holistic Approach for Seborrheic Dermatitis

Fewer Side Effects: Unlike pharmaceutical treatments, natural remedies and lifestyle adjustments typically have fewer side effects. This minimizes the risk of aggravating the condition or causing new issues.

Long-Term Healing: Holistic healing aims to restore the body's natural balance, which can lead to more sustainable, long-term relief from seborrheic dermatitis. It doesn't just mask symptoms but encourages the body to heal itself.

Improved Overall Health: Since holistic healing addresses the root causes of illness and promotes overall well-being, individuals often notice improvements in other areas of their health, such as better digestion, improved mood, and increased energy.

Seborrheic dermatitis can be a frustrating condition, but the holistic approach offers a comprehensive, natural way to manage and prevent its symptoms. By addressing the root causes — from diet and stress to gut health and environmental factors — holistic healing empowers individuals to take control of their health and improve their overall well-being. Through mindful living, natural remedies, and self-care practices, it is possible not only to alleviate seborrheic dermatitis but to thrive in a state of balance and vitality.

2.3 Integrating Body, Mind, and Skin Health
When we integrate body, mind, and skin health, we can promote natural healing and long-term

prevention of conditions like seborrheic dermatitis.

Understanding Seborrheic Dermatitis and Its Triggers

Before diving into a holistic approach, it's important to understand what may trigger seborrheic dermatitis. **The condition is often linked to:**

•Overactive sebaceous (oil-producing) glands

•Fungal overgrowth (specifically, a yeast called Malassezia).

•Inflammation.

•Weakened immune response.

While these are the physical factors, many patients also report flare-ups that are triggered by stress, lack of sleep, poor diet, and other lifestyle factors. This is where the holistic approach becomes valuable: it recognizes that treating the skin alone is not enough to achieve real healing.

The Three Pillars of Holistic Healing: Body, Mind, and Skin

The holistic approach to seborrheic dermatitis involves integrating care for the body, mind, and skin. **Let's explore each pillar:**

1. Body Health: Nourishing from Within

The body's internal health plays a crucial role in overall skin wellness. Here are some key aspects of maintaining body health to **prevent and heal seborrheic dermatitis:**

Diet and Nutrition:
A nutrient-rich diet supports skin health by providing the vitamins, minerals, and antioxidants needed for cellular repair and inflammation control. **Focus on:**

Omega-3 fatty acids (from sources like fish, flaxseeds, and walnuts) to reduce inflammation.

Probiotics and fermented foods (such as yogurt, kefir, and sauerkraut) to support gut health, which is closely linked to the immune system and skin.

Zinc and biotin for skin repair and maintaining proper oil production.

Vitamin D for immune system regulation.

Avoiding processed foods, excessive sugar, and dairy may also help reduce flare-ups, as these can trigger inflammation and worsen skin conditions.

Hydration:
Drinking plenty of water helps keep the skin hydrated and flushes out toxins that may contribute to irritation and dryness.

Exercise:

Regular physical activity improves circulation, which helps deliver oxygen and nutrients to the skin. Exercise also helps reduce stress, which is a known trigger for seborrheic dermatitis.

2. Mind Health: Managing Stress and Emotional Well-being

Stress is one of the most significant triggers of seborrheic dermatitis flare-ups. When we are stressed, our body releases hormones like cortisol that can increase inflammation and suppress immune function. **Focusing on mental health can have a profound impact on the skin:**

Mindfulness Practices:
Techniques like meditation, deep breathing exercises, and yoga help calm the nervous system and reduce the body's stress response. These practices encourage relaxation and mental clarity, which can help prevent stress-related skin issues.

Quality Sleep:
Sleep is when the body repairs itself, including the skin. Aim for seven to nine hours of uninterrupted sleep each night to support skin healing and overall health.

Emotional Balance:
Emotional health can affect physical health. Taking time for self-care, developing healthy routines, and seeking support for emotional challenges can improve mental well-being and reduce stress.

3. Skin Health: Gentle Care and Natural Remedies

While addressing internal factors is crucial, caring for the skin directly can help soothe symptoms and prevent flare-ups. A holistic approach to skin care emphasizes gentle, natural treatments:

Gentle Cleansing:

Over-cleansing or using harsh products can strip the skin of its natural oils and exacerbate seborrheic dermatitis. Opt for mild, sulfate-free cleansers that cleanse without irritating the skin.

Natural Moisturizers:
Moisturizing helps restore the skin's natural barrier. Look for products with natural **anti-inflammatory ingredients like:**

Aloe vera: Soothes irritation and reduces redness.

Coconut oil: Contains antifungal properties and helps retain moisture.

Tea tree oil: A natural antifungal essential oil that can help reduce Malassezia overgrowth when diluted properly.

Avoiding Triggers

Seborrheic dermatitis can be worsened by environmental factors like cold, dry weather or the use of alcohol-based skin products. Avoiding known triggers can help minimize flare-ups.

Sunlight Exposure:
Sunlight, in moderation, has been shown to improve seborrheic dermatitis symptoms. The ultraviolet (UV) light from the sun can reduce inflammation and help control yeast overgrowth on the skin. However, it's important to protect the skin from excessive sun exposure, as too much UV light can cause damage.

The Power of Integration: How It All Comes Together

Holistic healing is about recognizing that the skin is not an isolated organ but part of a larger system. By integrating care for the body, mind, and skin, we not only treat the symptoms of seborrheic dermatitis but also address its root causes. This approach promotes long-term healing and helps prevent future flare-ups.

While there is no one-size-fits-all solution, a holistic approach allows for personalized care. Each person's body, stress levels, and skin sensitivities are different, so it's important to listen to your body and adjust your routine as needed.

Seborrheic dermatitis can be a frustrating and persistent condition, but a holistic approach offers a path to healing that goes beyond temporary relief. By nourishing the body with a balanced diet, managing stress through mindfulness practices, and treating the skin with gentle, natural remedies, you can support your overall health and bring balance back to your skin.

Integrating body, mind, and skin health is not just about addressing symptoms—it's about creating a lifestyle that supports healing from the inside out. Through this comprehensive, thoughtful approach, you can achieve lasting relief and enjoy healthier skin for years to come.

Chapter 3

Diet and Nutrition for Healthy Skin

3.1 Anti-Inflammatory Foods

Seborrheic dermatitis can be managed and prevented through an anti-inflammatory diet. By incorporating foods that reduce inflammation and support skin health, you can naturally ease symptoms and promote healing. This guide provides clear, practical recipes with ingredients and instructions to help you nourish your skin from within.

Key Principles of an Anti-Inflammatory Diet

1. Focus on Whole Foods: Choose fresh, unprocessed foods to minimize exposure to additives and preservatives that may trigger inflammation.

2. Balance Omega Fatty Acids: Include omega-3-rich foods like fatty fish, flaxseeds, and walnuts while reducing omega-6 intake from processed oils.

3. Support Gut Health: Eat probiotic-rich foods like yogurt and fermented vegetables, and include prebiotic foods like garlic and onions to maintain a healthy gut microbiome.

4. Hydrate Well: Drink plenty of water and herbal teas to keep your skin hydrated and detoxified.

5. Minimize Trigger Foods: Avoid sugar, refined grains, dairy (if sensitive), alcohol, and fried foods that may worsen inflammation.

Recipes to Support Skin Health

1. Anti-Inflammatory Green Smoothie

This nutrient-packed smoothie is convenient to prepare and it's full of antioxidants.

Ingredients:

1 cup of unsweetened almond milk (alternatively, coconut water)

1 handful fresh spinach

1 small cucumber, peeled and chopped

1/2 avocado

1/2 green apple

1 tbsp ground flaxseed

1/2 tsp turmeric powder

Juice of 1/2 lemon

1/4 tsp black pepper (to enhance turmeric absorption)

4-5 ice cubes

Instructions:

1. Add all ingredients to a blender.

2. Blend until smooth and creamy.

3. Pour into a glass and enjoy immediately.

2. Salmon and Quinoa Salad

A perfect balance of omega-3 fatty acids, antioxidants, and fiber.

Ingredients:

1 cup cooked quinoa

4 oz grilled salmon

1 cup mixed greens (spinach, arugula, kale)

1/4 cup cherry tomatoes, halved

1/4 avocado, sliced

1 tbsp olive oil

1 tsp apple cider vinegar

1/4 tsp sea salt

1/4 tsp black pepper

Instructions:

1. Prepare the quinoa according to package instructions and let it cool.

2. Grill or bake salmon until fully cooked.

3. In a large bowl, combine quinoa, mixed greens, cherry tomatoes, and avocado.

4. Flake the salmon over the salad.

5. Drizzle with olive oil and apple cider vinegar, then season with salt and pepper. Toss gently and serve.

3. Golden Turmeric Latte

This anti-inflammatory drink is soothing and perfect for calming the skin from within.

Ingredients:

1 cup unsweetened almond milk

1/2 tsp turmeric powder

1/4 tsp ground cinnamon

1/4 tsp ginger powder

1 tsp honey or maple syrup (optional)

Pinch of black pepper

Instructions:

1. Heat the almond milk in a small saucepan over medium heat.

2. Whisk in turmeric, cinnamon, ginger, and black pepper.

3. Allow to simmer for 2-3 minutes, then remove from heat.

4. Sweeten with honey or maple syrup if desired.

5. Transfer to a mug and savor it while it's warm.

4. Roasted Sweet Potatoes with Garlic and Herbs

Rich in beta-carotene and antioxidants, this dish supports skin repair.

Ingredients:

2 medium sweet potatoes, cubed

2 tbsp olive oil

2 cloves garlic, minced

1 tsp dried rosemary

1/2 tsp smoked paprika

1/4 tsp sea salt

Instructions:

1. Preheat your oven to 400°F (200°C).

2. Toss the sweet potato cubes with olive oil, garlic, rosemary, paprika, and salt.

3. Spread evenly on a baking sheet lined with parchment paper.

4. Roast for 25-30 minutes, flipping halfway through, until tender and golden.

5. Blueberry Chia Pudding

A simple, antioxidant-rich breakfast or snack to reduce inflammation.

Ingredients:

1/2 cup unsweetened almond milk

3 tbsp chia seeds

1/4 tsp vanilla extract

1/2 cup fresh blueberries

1 tsp honey (optional)

Instructions:

1. In a bowl or jar, blend together almond milk, chia seeds, and vanilla extract.

2. Stir well to prevent clumping and let sit for 5 minutes. Stir again.

3. Seal the container and refrigerate for a minimum of 2 hours or overnight.

4. Top with fresh blueberries and a drizzle of honey before serving.

Daily Tips for Success

Plan Your Meals: Prep your ingredients ahead to make healthy eating convenient.

Stay Consistent: Stick to the diet to see long-term improvements.

Monitor Skin Health: Track how your skin reacts to different foods.

By focusing on an anti-inflammatory diet, you can nourish your skin, reduce flare-ups, and improve overall health naturally.

3.2 Gut Health and Skin Connection

While the exact cause of Seborrheic dermatitis is not fully understood, research suggests that the health of your gut plays a vital role in its onset, severity, and management.

Understanding The Gut-skin Axis

The gut-skin axis refers to the two-way communication between the gastrointestinal system and the skin. The balance of bacteria in the gut, also known as the gut microbiome, affects inflammation, immune responses, and overall skin health. When the gut microbiome is disrupted, it can lead to systemic inflammation, which may trigger or worsen seborrheic dermatitis.

Key Gut Health Factors Affecting Seborrheic Dermatitis

1. Microbiome Imbalance (Dysbiosis):
A lack of beneficial bacteria can compromise the gut lining, allowing toxins and inflammatory substances to enter the bloodstream and impact skin health.

2. Inflammation and Immune Response:

An unhealthy gut often leads to chronic low-grade inflammation, which can worsen skin conditions, including seborrheic dermatitis.

3. Dietary Influences:
Poor dietary choices, such as consuming excess sugar, processed foods, and unhealthy fats, can feed harmful gut bacteria and exacerbate inflammation.

Natural Healing Strategies for Gut and Skin Health

1. Adopt a Gut-Friendly Diet:

Focus on Whole Foods: Include plenty of vegetables, fruits, whole grains, and lean proteins. These provide fiber and nutrients that support a healthy microbiome.

Incorporate Fermented Foods: Yogurt, kefir, sauerkraut, and kimchi are rich in probiotics that restore beneficial gut bacteria.

Limit Sugars and Processed Foods: These can disrupt the microbiome and increase inflammation.

2. Consider Prebiotics and Probiotics:

Prebiotics, found in foods like garlic, onions, and bananas, feed healthy gut bacteria. Probiotics, available in fermented foods or supplements, introduce beneficial bacteria.

3. Support Digestive Health:

Drink plenty of water to aid digestion and toxin removal.

Include digestive enzymes or apple cider vinegar before meals to enhance nutrient absorption.

4. Address Food Sensitivities:

Gluten, dairy, or other allergens may contribute to gut inflammation. Keeping a food journal can help identify and eliminate triggers.

5. Manage Stress:

Persistent stress can interfere with digestive processes and immune system stability. Practices like mindfulness, yoga, and deep breathing can help reduce stress-related inflammation.

6. Promote Regular Detoxification:

Liver Support: Eat cruciferous vegetables (e.g., broccoli, cauliflower) to enhance liver detoxification.

Hydration: Ensure adequate water intake to flush out toxins.

Preventing Seborrheic Dermatitis Through Gut Health

1. Maintain a Balanced Diet: Regularly consuming nutrient-rich and anti-inflammatory foods ensures a healthy microbiome.

2. Stay Active: Exercise improves gut motility and supports a healthy immune response.

3. Avoid Harsh Products: Gentle skincare combined with a balanced gut environment reduces flare-ups.

4. Monitor Lifestyle Changes: Track what works for you to maintain consistency in diet, stress management, and skincare practices.

By focusing on the connection between gut health and skin, individuals can take meaningful steps to naturally heal and prevent seborrheic dermatitis. A holistic approach that combines diet, lifestyle, and mindfulness supports not only clearer skin but also overall well-being.

3.3 Foods to Avoid for Flare Prevention

Seborrheic dermatitis is a chronic skin condition often influenced by diet, lifestyle, and overall health. While it is not caused solely by food, certain dietary choices can exacerbate inflammation, trigger flare-ups, or weaken the skin's natural defenses. Avoiding these foods can help manage symptoms and support your body's natural healing process.

1. Refined Sugars and Processed Sweets

Excess sugar in the diet promotes inflammation throughout the body. It can also disrupt your gut microbiome, weakening your skin's natural barrier and contributing to flare-ups.

Examples to avoid:

- Sodas, candies, and pastries.

- Sweetened cereals and flavored yogurts.

- High-fructose corn syrup in packaged foods.

2. Dairy Products

For some individuals, dairy products can worsen seborrheic dermatitis. Dairy can stimulate excess oil production and potentially trigger an inflammatory response in sensitive individuals.

Examples to avoid:

•Milk, cream, and butter.

•Cheese, ice cream, and yogurt.

3. Gluten and Refined Grains

Highly processed grains and gluten-containing foods may aggravate inflammation or trigger sensitivity in some people, particularly if they have gluten intolerance or leaky gut syndrome.

Examples to avoid:

•White bread and pasta.

•Baked goods made with refined flour.

•Processed snacks like crackers and pretzels.

4. Fried and Greasy Foods

Foods high in unhealthy fats can increase oil production on the skin, which may worsen seborrheic dermatitis symptoms. Trans fats and saturated fats, in particular, should be avoided.

Examples to avoid:

- Deep-fried foods (e.g., french fries, fried chicken).

- Processed snacks like chips and packaged baked goods.

- Fast foods and heavily buttered dishes.

5. Alcohol

Alcohol consumption can dehydrate the skin and weaken its natural defenses. Additionally, alcohol can disrupt gut health and impair the liver's ability to process toxins, potentially contributing to flare-ups.

Examples to avoid:

- Beer, wine, and spirits.

- Cocktails with high sugar content.

6. Spicy Foods

Spicy foods can cause skin irritation and worsen inflammation in sensitive individuals. For some, they also trigger sweating, which may aggravate seborrheic dermatitis symptoms.

Examples to avoid:

- Hot peppers and chili-based sauces.

- Spiced curries and stir-fried dishes with excessive heat.

7. High-Histamine Foods

Foods high in histamines or those that trigger histamine release can aggravate seborrheic dermatitis in some individuals prone to histamine intolerance.

Examples to avoid:

- Aged cheeses and fermented products (e.g., sauerkraut, soy sauce).

- Smoked meats and fish.

- Certain fruits like bananas and avocados.

8. Artificial Additives and Preservatives

Many processed foods contain artificial colors, flavors, and preservatives that can irritate the skin or trigger inflammation.

Examples to avoid:

- Packaged snacks, frozen meals, and instant noodles.

•Sodas and artificially flavored beverages.

•Foods with long ingredient lists containing unfamiliar chemicals.

A Holistic Approach

While avoiding these foods can help prevent flare-ups, it's equally important to focus on nutrient-dense, anti-inflammatory foods that support gut health and strengthen the skin barrier. Drinking plenty of water, reducing stress, and maintaining a balanced lifestyle also play vital roles in managing seborrheic dermatitis.

Chapter 4

Natural Remedies and Topical Solutions

4.1 Essential Oils and Herbal Treatments

Natural remedies involving essential oils and herbal treatments offer gentle yet effective ways to manage and prevent flare-ups. Below are detailed recipes for natural remedies, along with clear instructions and ingredients.

1. Tea Tree Oil Scalp Treatment

Purpose: Reduce inflammation, control dandruff, and combat fungal overgrowth.

Ingredients:

5 drops of tea tree essential oil

2 tablespoons of coconut oil (carrier oil)

Instructions:

1. Mix the tea tree essential oil and coconut oil in a small bowl.

2. Gently massage the mixture into your scalp, focusing on affected areas.

3. Leave it on for at least 30 minutes or overnight for deeper absorption.

4. Rinse thoroughly with a mild shampoo.

5. Repeat 2–3 times a week.

2. Aloe Vera and Lavender Soothing Gel

Purpose: Soothe irritation, reduce redness, and moisturize the skin.

Ingredients:

2 tablespoons of fresh aloe vera gel

3 drops of lavender essential oil

Instructions:

1. Combine aloe vera gel and lavender oil in a clean container.

2. Apply a thin layer of the mixture to the affected skin areas.

3. Allow it to absorb fully—do not rinse.

4. Use twice daily, morning and evening.

3. Chamomile and Calendula Herbal Wash

Purpose: Calm inflamed skin and promote healing.

Ingredients:

1 tablespoon of dried chamomile flowers

1 tablespoon of dried calendula petals

2 cups of water

Instructions:

1. Bring water to a boil, then add chamomile and calendula.

2. Cover and steep for 10–15 minutes.

3. Strain the liquid and let it cool.

4. Use a cotton pad to gently apply the herbal wash to affected areas or rinse the scalp.

5. Use daily for best results.

4. Neem Oil and Rosemary Treatment

Purpose: Fight fungal growth and improve scalp circulation.

Ingredients:

1 teaspoon of neem oil

4 drops of rosemary essential oil

2 tablespoons of jojoba oil (carrier oil)

Instructions:

1. Blend all ingredients in a small bowl.

2. Massage the mixture onto your scalp or skin.

3. Leave it on for 30 minutes, then rinse with lukewarm water and a gentle cleanser or shampoo.

4. Repeat 2–3 times a week.

5. Apple Cider Vinegar Herbal Rinse

Purpose: Restore the skin's pH balance and reduce flakes.

Ingredients:

2 tablespoons of apple cider vinegar

1 cup of water

1 teaspoon of dried rosemary or thyme

Instructions:

1. Steep the dried herb in hot water for 10 minutes, then strain.

2. Mix the herbal infusion with apple cider vinegar.

3. After washing your hair, pour the rinse over your scalp and let it sit for 5–10 minutes.

4. Rinse with lukewarm water.

5. Use 2–3 times a week.

6. Turmeric and Honey Mask

Purpose: Reduce inflammation and moisturize the skin.

Ingredients:

1 teaspoon of turmeric powder

1 tablespoon of raw honey

1–2 teaspoons of yogurt (optional for added hydration)

Instructions:

1. Mix turmeric and honey (and yogurt, if desired) into a paste.

2. Apply a thin layer to the affected areas.

3. Leave it on for 15–20 minutes.

4. Rinse gently with warm water.

5. Use 2–3 times a week.

General Tips:

•Always do a patch test before using any new remedy to ensure no allergic reactions.

•Use organic, high-quality ingredients to maximize effectiveness.

•Maintain consistent use for at least 2–4 weeks to observe noticeable improvements.

These natural solutions not only target the symptoms of seborrheic dermatitis but also help improve overall skin health. With patience and regular application, these treatments can provide relief and promote long-term prevention.

4.2 DIY Natural Skincare Recipes

Seborrheic dermatitis, characterized by redness, flaking, and itching, can often be managed with natural remedies that support skin healing and balance. Below are simple, effective DIY skincare recipes to help soothe and prevent flare-ups.

1. Calming Aloe Vera and Tea Tree Oil Gel

Purpose: Reduces inflammation and itching while combating fungal overgrowth.

Ingredients:

2 tablespoons fresh aloe vera gel (pure, organic)

2 drops tea tree essential oil

1 teaspoon coconut oil (optional, if your skin tolerates it)

Instructions:

1. Scoop out fresh aloe vera gel from a leaf and place it in a clean bowl.

2. Combine the tea tree oil in the mixture and stir thoroughly. If using coconut oil, melt it slightly and stir it into the mixture.

3. Apply a thin layer to the affected areas, avoiding the eyes.

4. Allow it to sit for 20 minutes, then rinse thoroughly with warm water.

5. Use daily for best results.

2. Soothing Oatmeal and Honey Mask

Purpose: Hydrates and calms irritated skin while promoting healing.

Ingredients:

2 tablespoons finely ground oats (colloidal oatmeal works best)

1 tablespoon raw honey

1-2 tablespoons warm water

Instructions:

1. Mix the ground oats and honey in a small bowl.

2. Add warm water a little at a time to form a paste.

3. Apply the mask to clean, damp skin, focusing on affected areas.

4. Let it sit for 15–20 minutes, then rinse off gently with lukewarm water.

5. Use 2–3 times a week to reduce redness and flaking.

3. Apple Cider Vinegar Rinse

Purpose: Balances skin pH and reduces fungal growth.

Ingredients:

1/4 cup raw, unfiltered apple cider vinegar

1/2 cup distilled water

Instructions:

1. Mix the apple cider vinegar and water in a clean container.

2. Apply the mixture to the scalp or affected areas with a cotton ball or spray bottle.

3. Leave it on for 10–15 minutes, then rinse thoroughly with cool water.

4. Use 1–2 times weekly, adjusting frequency based on skin tolerance.

4. Gentle Coconut Oil and Lavender Balm

Purpose: Moisturizes and calms itchy, dry patches.

Ingredients:

2 tablespoons organic virgin coconut oil

3 drops lavender essential oil

Instructions:

1. Melt the coconut oil gently in a double boiler or microwave.

2. Stir in the lavender oil until well blended.

3. Let the mixture cool slightly, then apply to dry patches.

4. Use at night as an overnight moisturizer.

5. Chamomile and Calendula Compress

Purpose: Reduces redness and soothes irritated skin.

Ingredients:

1 tablespoon dried chamomile flowers

1 tablespoon dried calendula flowers

1 cup boiling water

Instructions:

1. Add the chamomile and calendula flowers to a cup of boiling water.

2. Steep for 10 minutes, then strain and let the tea cool slightly.

3. Soak a clean cloth or cotton pad in the infusion and apply it to affected areas.

4. Maintain the compress in place for a duration of 10 to 15 minutes.

5. Repeat daily for calming relief.

6. Nourishing Avocado and Yogurt Mask

Purpose: Hydrates and provides probiotics to balance the skin's microbiome.

Ingredients:

1/2 ripe avocado

2 tablespoons plain, unsweetened yogurt

Instructions:
1. In a bowl, thoroughly mash the avocado until it reaches a creamy consistency.

2. Mix in the yogurt until well combined.

3. Apply the mask to clean skin, avoiding the eyes.

4. Leave it on for 15 minutes, then rinse off with lukewarm water.

5. Use weekly to maintain hydrated, balanced skin.

7. DIY Anti-Fungal Herbal Oil Blend

Purpose: Targets fungal overgrowth that may trigger seborrheic dermatitis.

Ingredients:

2 tablespoons jojoba oil or olive oil

2 drops tea tree essential oil

2 drops rosemary essential oil

1 drop neem oil

Instructions:

1. Combine all oils in a small glass bottle. Shake well.

2. Apply a few drops to affected areas and massage gently.

3. Leave it on for at least 30 minutes before washing off or leave overnight if tolerated.

4. Use 2–3 times a week.

Tips for Success

Patch Test First: Always test new remedies on a small area of skin to ensure no adverse reactions.

Be Consistent: Frequently, natural treatments require a certain amount of time to display their outcomes. Maintain a routine for some weeks.

Avoid Triggers: Manage stress, eat a healthy diet, and avoid harsh skincare products.

Consult a Dermatologist: If symptoms persist or worsen, seek professional advice.

These recipes are designed to gently soothe and support your skin's natural healing process. Regular care, combined with healthy lifestyle choices, can significantly improve seborrheic dermatitis symptoms.

4.3 Safe and Effective Over-the-Counter Options

Seborrheic dermatitis can often be managed effectively with safe, natural over-the-counter remedies. These solutions not only target symptoms but also address the underlying triggers, such as inflammation, excess oil production, and microbial imbalances. Below is a comprehensive guide to natural remedies and topical solutions that can support the healing and prevention of this condition.

1. Tea Tree Oil-Based Products

Tea tree oil, derived from the leaves of the Melaleuca alternifolia plant, is well-known for its antifungal and anti-inflammatory properties. Many over-the-counter shampoos and creams contain diluted tea tree oil to help control Malassezia yeast, a common trigger of seborrheic dermatitis.

How to Use: Look for a shampoo with 2–5% tea tree oil. Use it 2–3 times per week, leaving it on the scalp for a few minutes before rinsing. For skin, dilute a few drops of tea tree oil in a carrier oil (such as coconut or jojoba) and apply it sparingly to affected areas.

2. Aloe Vera Gel

Aloe vera is a natural anti-inflammatory and soothing agent that can reduce redness and itching. It also promotes healing by hydrating the skin and restoring its natural barrier.

How to Use: Choose 100% pure aloe vera gel without added chemicals or fragrances. Spread a light coating on clean, dry skin two times a day.

3. Apple Cider Vinegar (ACV)

Apple cider vinegar's natural acidity can help balance the skin's pH and reduce fungal overgrowth. It also acts as a gentle exfoliant to remove flakes and dead skin cells.

How to Use: Combine the same amount of apple cider vinegar and water. Using a cotton ball, dab the solution onto affected areas or use it as a rinse for the scalp after shampooing. Don't apply undiluted ACV so as to avoid irritation.

4. Coconut Oil

Coconut oil is rich in medium-chain fatty acids with antimicrobial and moisturizing properties. It can soothe irritation, reduce inflammation, and restore moisture to dry, flaky skin.

How to Use: Warm a small amount of virgin coconut oil and gently massage it into the scalp or affected skin. Leave it on for 30 minutes or overnight, then rinse with a gentle cleanser.

5. Honey Masks

Raw honey has powerful antifungal and anti-inflammatory effects. It also provides deep hydration, which can help alleviate dryness and flaking.

How to Use: Mix 1–2 tablespoons of raw honey with a few drops of water to create a spreadable paste. Spread it over the affected regions, allow it to sit for 20 minutes, and then rinse off with lukewarm water. Apply this remedy 1 to 2 times every week.

6. Probiotic Skincare

Probiotics, commonly associated with gut health, can also benefit the skin by promoting a balanced microbiome. Over-the-counter creams and serums containing probiotics can reduce inflammation and prevent yeast overgrowth.

How to Use: Apply probiotic-infused skincare products as directed on the packaging, usually once or twice daily on clean skin.

7. Colloidal Oatmeal

Colloidal oatmeal is a finely ground form of oats known for its soothing and anti-inflammatory properties. It alleviates itching, redness, and irritation.

How to Use: Look for creams or lotions with colloidal oatmeal as an active ingredient. Apply liberally to freshly cleansed skin as required to ease discomfort.

8. Zinc Pyrithione Shampoos and Creams

Zinc pyrithione possesses antifungal and antibacterial characteristics that aid in managing Malassezia yeast and alleviating inflammation. It is gentle enough for regular use on the scalp or skin.

How to Use: Choose a zinc pyrithione shampoo and use it 2–3 times weekly. For skin, apply zinc-based creams to affected areas once or twice daily.

9. Calendula Cream

Calendula, or marigold extract, is a natural anti-inflammatory and antifungal agent that soothes irritated skin and reduces redness.

How to Use: Apply calendula cream to clean, dry skin 2–3 times daily. Choose products free from synthetic fragrances or preservatives.

10. Natural Salicylic Acid Treatments

Salicylic acid, derived from willow bark, gently exfoliates the skin and removes scales associated with seborrheic dermatitis. It also helps reduce clogged pores and inflammation.

How to Use: Use a salicylic acid-based shampoo or cream 1–2 times per week. Refrain from using it too frequently to avoid causing excessive dryness or irritation.

While these natural over-the-counter remedies are generally safe, patch-testing new products is essential to rule out allergic reactions or sensitivities. Consistent use, combined with a healthy lifestyle, can significantly improve seborrheic dermatitis symptoms. Always consult a dermatologist for severe or persistent cases to ensure a tailored treatment plan.

Chapter 5

Stress Management and Emotional Well-Being

5.1 The Stress-Skin Connection

Seborrheic dermatitis can be significantly influenced by stress. While the root causes of this condition often include genetic predispositions, fungal imbalances, and inflammation, stress plays a key role in triggering or worsening symptoms. Understanding the stress-skin connection and adopting effective stress management techniques can be transformative for healing and prevention.

How Stress Affects Skin Health

Stress activates the body's fight-or-flight response, releasing hormones such as cortisol. While this response is natural and useful in short-term situations, chronic stress can lead to prolonged elevation of cortisol levels. **This disrupts the body's balance in several ways:**

1. Weakened Skin Barrier: Chronic stress impairs the skin's ability to retain moisture and fend off external irritants. This can make the skin more vulnerable to seborrheic dermatitis flare-ups.

2. Increased Inflammation: Stress amplifies inflammatory responses in the body, worsening conditions like redness and scaling associated with seborrheic dermatitis.

3. Impaired Immune Function: A stressed immune system is less effective at regulating fungal growth, such as Malassezia, which is often linked to seborrheic dermatitis.

The Mind-Skin Loop

Stress not only affects the skin, but visible skin conditions like seborrheic dermatitis can also contribute to emotional distress. This creates a feedback loop where stress worsens the condition, and the condition intensifies stress. Breaking this cycle is crucial for long-term healing.

Practical Stress Management Techniques

To manage stress and support your skin's healing process, adopt these proven strategies:

1. Mindfulness and Meditation:

Practice mindfulness techniques to calm your mind and regulate stress. Even 10 minutes of deep breathing or guided meditation daily can reduce cortisol levels.

Techniques like progressive muscle relaxation can ease physical tension that contributes to stress.

2. Physical Activity:

Exercise reduces stress hormones while increasing endorphins, the body's natural mood boosters. Gentle activities like yoga, tai chi, or walking are particularly effective for stress-related skin issues.

3. Quality Sleep:

Sleep is a natural reset for the body and mind. Aim for 7-9 hours of quality sleep each night to help the skin repair and regenerate. Create a soothing nighttime ritual to enhance your sleep quality.

4. Journaling and Emotional Expression:

Write down your thoughts and feelings to process stress in a healthy way. Journaling can clarify problems, reduce anxiety, and improve your sense of control.

5. Social Connection:

Share your experiences with trusted friends or support groups. Talking about stress can ease its burden and help you gain perspective.

6. Balanced Nutrition and Hydration:

Stress often leads to poor dietary choices. Focus on whole, nutrient-dense foods that support gut health and reduce inflammation, such as leafy greens, nuts, and omega-3-rich fish. Stay hydrated to maintain skin elasticity and moisture.

7. Set Boundaries and Prioritize Self-Care:

Learn to say no to unnecessary stressors and set aside time for relaxation and activities that bring you joy.

Emotional Well-Being and Skin Health

Emotional well-being is just as important as physical care in managing seborrheic dermatitis. Addressing underlying emotional challenges, such as anxiety or unresolved conflicts, can prevent stress from escalating. Practices such as gratitude journaling, engaging in hobbies, and seeking therapy when needed all contribute to a balanced and positive mindset.

Long-Term Benefits of Stress Management

Consistent stress management not only improves seborrheic dermatitis but also enhances overall skin health. By regulating stress, you create an environment in which your body can heal naturally. Skin becomes less reactive, and inflammatory conditions like seborrheic dermatitis become less frequent and severe.

The stress-skin connection is a powerful reminder of the importance of holistic well-being. Managing stress and nurturing emotional health are key steps in the natural healing and prevention of seborrheic dermatitis. By taking small but meaningful actions each day, you can break the stress cycle and support your skin in its journey to health and vitality.

5.2 Mindfulness, Meditation, and Relaxation Techniques

Seborrheic dermatitis, a chronic skin condition, often has underlying triggers related to stress and emotional imbalance. While addressing physical causes is crucial, focusing on mental and emotional well-being can significantly improve healing and prevent flare-ups. Mindfulness, meditation, and relaxation techniques are powerful tools for managing stress and supporting overall health, including skin health.

Understanding the Connection Between Stress and Seborrheic Dermatitis

Stress triggers the release of hormones like cortisol, which can disrupt the immune system and increase inflammation in the body. For individuals with seborrheic dermatitis, this can worsen symptoms like redness, scaling, and irritation. By reducing stress, you not only help your body maintain balance but also support your skin's natural healing process.

Mindfulness for Emotional Balance

Mindfulness is the practice of being present and fully engaged in the moment without judgment. It helps calm the mind, reduce stress, and improve emotional regulation.

Steps to Practice Mindfulness:

1. Set aside time: Start with 5–10 minutes daily. Gradually increase as you become more comfortable.

2. Focus on your breath: Sit quietly and take slow, deep breaths. Pay attention to the sensation of air entering and leaving your nostrils.

3. Notice your thoughts: Allow thoughts to come and go without clinging to them. Return your focus to your breath if your mind wanders.

4. Engage your senses: During daily activities, notice the sights, sounds, smells, and textures around you. This anchors you to the present moment.

Benefits for Skin Health:

•Lowers cortisol levels, reducing inflammation.

•Improves sleep quality, aiding skin repair.

•Creates a sense of calm, which helps break the stress-skin cycle.

Meditation for Relaxation and Healing

Meditation is a structured practice that promotes relaxation and enhances self-awareness. It trains your mind to stay calm and focused, which can positively impact your overall health.

Simple Meditation Techniques:

1. Body Scan Meditation

•Lie down in a quiet space.

- Close your eyes and take slow, deep breaths.

- Focus on each part of your body, starting from your toes and moving up to your head.

- Notice any tension and consciously relax those areas.

2. Guided Imagery Meditation

- Sit or lie down in a peaceful spot.

- Visualize a calming scene, such as a beach or a forest.

- Imagine the sights, sounds, and sensations of this place.

- Let this imagery soothe your mind and body.

3. Loving-Kindness Meditation

- Sit comfortably and breathe deeply.

- Silently repeat phrases like "May I be happy, may I be healthy, may I live with ease."

- Extend these wishes to others, including those you love and even people who challenge you.

Benefits for Seborrheic Dermatitis:

- Enhances blood flow, promoting skin repair.

- Reduces anxiety, a common trigger for flare-ups.

- Supports hormonal balance, leading to healthier skin.

Relaxation Techniques for Stress Relief

Incorporating relaxation into your daily routine helps your body recover from stress and prevents it from becoming chronic.

Effective Relaxation Techniques:

1. Progressive Muscle Relaxation (PMR)

• Sit or lie down comfortably.

• Tense each muscle group (e.g., feet, legs, arms) for 5 seconds, then release.

• Notice the feeling of relaxation spreading through your body.

2. Deep Breathing Exercises

• Inhale deeply through your nose for a count of 4.

• Hold the breath for 4 counts.

• Exhale slowly through your mouth for a count of 6.

• Repeat for 5–10 minutes.

3. Aromatherapy

Use calming essential oils like lavender or chamomile in a diffuser.

Inhale deeply to promote relaxation and improve mood.

4. Yoga or Tai Chi

These practices combine gentle movements with controlled breathing.

They release physical tension and calm the mind.

Creating a Daily Practice for Long-Term Benefits

Consistency is key to reaping the benefits of mindfulness, meditation, and relaxation. **Here's a simple plan to integrate these techniques into your life:**

Morning: Start your day with 5 minutes of deep breathing or body scan meditation to set a positive tone.

Midday: Take short mindfulness breaks. Focus on your breath or surroundings for a few minutes.

Evening: Wind down with a guided imagery meditation or progressive muscle relaxation. Pair this with aromatherapy for added benefits.

The Role of Emotional Resilience in Healing

Developing emotional resilience helps you navigate life's challenges without letting stress overwhelm you. Regular mindfulness and meditation practices strengthen this resilience, helping you maintain balance even in difficult times.

While seborrheic dermatitis can be physically and emotionally challenging, managing stress through mindfulness, meditation, and relaxation techniques is a holistic and empowering way to support healing. By calming your mind and reducing stress, you create an environment where your body—and your skin—can thrive. Consistent practice not only improves your skin but also enhances your overall quality of life.

5.3 Creating a Balanced Lifestyle for Skin Health

Seborrheic dermatitis is a common skin condition influenced by a mix of internal and external factors. Stress and emotional imbalances are known triggers, making it vital to adopt a balanced lifestyle that supports both mental and physical health. Here, we explore how managing stress and nurturing emotional well-being can help prevent and heal seborrheic dermatitis naturally.

Understanding the Stress-Skin Connection

Stress has a profound effect on the body. It weakens the immune system, disrupts hormone levels, and exacerbates inflammatory responses—all of which can trigger or worsen seborrheic dermatitis. Chronic stress also contributes to poor sleep, unhealthy eating habits, and a lack of self-care, further aggravating skin issues.

The skin acts as a mirror, reflecting internal struggles. Emotional imbalances like anxiety, anger, or sadness can manifest as flare-ups, making stress management a cornerstone in natural healing.

Practical Stress Management Techniques

1. Daily Mindfulness Practices
Mindfulness helps calm the mind and reduce stress. Techniques like deep breathing, meditation, or even a simple five-minute body scan can lower cortisol levels, the stress hormone linked to inflammation. Begin your day with mindful breathing to set a peaceful tone and end it with gratitude journaling to focus on the positive aspects of your life.

2. Regular Exercise for Emotional Balance

Physical activity releases endorphins, the body's natural "feel-good" chemicals. Opt for moderate activities such as walking, yoga, or tai chi, which not only reduce stress but also improve circulation, aiding skin repair and renewal.

3. Healthy Sleep Habits

Sleep is a powerful healer. Poor sleep increases stress and inflammation. Aim for 7–9 hours of restful sleep each night by creating a calming bedtime routine—dim the lights, limit screen time, and consider herbal teas like chamomile to relax your mind.

4. Balanced Nutrition

A diet rich in anti-inflammatory foods can reduce stress and promote skin health. Incorporate omega-3 fatty acids, found in salmon and walnuts, and antioxidant-rich fruits and vegetables to fight inflammation. Avoid high-sugar and processed foods that can exacerbate stress and skin conditions.

5. Time in Nature
Spending time outdoors in green spaces or engaging in grounding activities, such as walking barefoot on grass, reduces cortisol levels and enhances emotional well-being. Natural sunlight can also provide a boost of vitamin D, essential for healthy skin.

6. Journaling and Emotional Expression
Writing down your thoughts and emotions can provide clarity and relief. Explore your feelings in a journal, or talk openly with trusted friends or a therapist. Suppressing emotions can lead to physical manifestations, including skin flare-ups.

7. Limit Stressors
Identify and minimize avoidable stressors in your daily routine. Simplify your schedule, delegate tasks, and practice saying "no" when overwhelmed. Balance your responsibilities with downtime to recharge.

Cultivating Emotional Well-Being

1. Develop a Support Network

Surround yourself with positive, understanding people who uplift your spirit. Regular social interactions can help reduce feelings of isolation, which often contribute to stress.

2. Practice Self-Compassion

Be kind to yourself. Accept that healing takes time and that setbacks are part of the process. Replace self-criticism with encouraging self-talk to reduce emotional stress.

3. Engage in Creative Activities

Art, music, and other creative outlets help release pent-up emotions and reduce stress. Painting, playing an instrument, or even gardening can provide joy and relaxation, nurturing emotional health.

4. Learn to Let Go

Practice forgiveness and let go of past grudges. Carrying emotional burdens increases stress, while forgiveness fosters peace and emotional resilience.

The Role of Consistency and Patience

Creating a balanced lifestyle requires consistent effort. Changes won't happen overnight, but small, daily actions add up to significant improvements in your skin and overall well-being. By prioritizing stress management and emotional health, you empower your body's natural ability to heal and prevent seborrheic dermatitis.

Your skin thrives when your mind and body are in harmony. Stress management and emotional well-being are not just supportive measures—they are essential tools for natural healing and prevention. Commit to a balanced lifestyle, and you'll not only see the difference in your skin but also feel the transformation in your entire life.

Chapter 6

Detoxifying Your Environment

6.1 Identifying Harmful Chemicals and Irritants

Seborrheic dermatitis is a persistent skin condition that can be aggravated by exposure to harmful chemicals and irritants. Detoxifying your environment can play a crucial role in both preventing flare-ups and promoting natural healing. By identifying and eliminating these irritants, you create a healthier, less inflammatory environment for your skin.

1. Common Household Irritants

Everyday household items often contain chemicals that can worsen seborrheic dermatitis. **Look out for:**

Harsh Cleaning Products: Many detergents, disinfectants, and sprays contain chemicals like ammonia, bleach, and synthetic fragrances that can irritate sensitive skin. Opt for natural alternatives, such as vinegar, baking soda, or unscented, eco-friendly cleaning products.

Synthetic Air Fresheners: Plug-ins, sprays, and scented candles may release volatile organic compounds (VOCs), which can irritate the skin and respiratory system. Replace these with essential oils or potpourri.

2. Personal Care Products to Avoid

Skin and hair products often include ingredients that trigger irritation:

Sodium Lauryl Sulfate (SLS): Found in shampoos and body washes, this harsh surfactant can strip natural oils and disrupt the skin barrier. Use sulfate-free products instead.

Synthetic Fragrances and Dyes: These are common in lotions, creams, and cosmetics.

Choose fragrance-free and dye-free alternatives labeled "for sensitive skin."

Alcohol-Based Products: Often used in toners or cleansers, alcohol can dry out the skin, worsening inflammation. Look for alcohol-free formulations.

3. Environmental Toxins

Indoor and outdoor pollution can also contribute to seborrheic dermatitis:

Dust and Mold: Allergens like dust mites and mold spores can irritate the skin. Clean your home regularly, use a dehumidifier, and address water leaks promptly to prevent mold growth.

Chemical Pesticides and Herbicides: Avoid using these in your garden or around your home. Opt for natural pest control methods, such as neem oil or diatomaceous earth.

4. Detoxifying Your Environment

Here's how to create a safer, cleaner space for your skin:

Switch to Natural Alternatives: Replace synthetic products with organic or homemade options. For example, use coconut oil as a moisturizer or apple cider vinegar as a gentle cleanser.

Improve Air Quality: Invest in an air purifier to remove airborne irritants. Regularly ventilate your home by opening windows when possible.

Check Your Water Source: Hard water or water treated with high levels of chlorine can irritate sensitive skin. Consider installing a water softener or a filter for your showerhead.

5. Diet and Hydration

While this focuses on external irritants, remember that what you consume affects your skin. Avoid processed foods high in preservatives and additives, as they may exacerbate inflammation. Stay hydrated to keep your skin healthy from the inside out.

6. Monitoring and Adjusting

Take note of how your skin responds to different products and environmental factors. Keeping a journal can help you identify and eliminate specific irritants that may trigger flare-ups.

By detoxifying your environment and adopting a natural approach, you reduce the risk of irritants aggravating seborrheic dermatitis. This thoughtful, proactive strategy not only supports healthier skin but also fosters overall well-being.

6.2 Switching to Natural Skincare and Household Products

Seborrheic dermatitis is often aggravated by environmental toxins and harsh chemicals in personal care and household products. Transitioning to natural alternatives can reduce exposure to irritants, support skin healing, and create a healthier overall environment. This shift not only benefits your skin but also contributes to a toxin-free home.

Understanding the Problem

Many conventional skincare and household products contain synthetic ingredients, fragrances, and preservatives that can disrupt the skin's natural barrier and worsen seborrheic dermatitis symptoms.

Common culprits include:

Sodium lauryl sulfate (SLS): Found in soaps and shampoos, it can strip the skin of natural oils.

Parabens: Used as preservatives, they may trigger irritation in sensitive skin.

Synthetic fragrances: Often composed of unknown chemicals, they can exacerbate inflammation.

Benefits of Natural Alternatives

Switching to natural products eliminates these harmful substances, allowing the skin to recover without constant exposure to irritants. Natural products often incorporate ingredients with healing and soothing properties, such as aloe vera, chamomile, and coconut oil.

Steps to Detoxify Your Skincare Routine

1. Evaluate Your Current Products: Read ingredient labels and identify items with potentially harmful chemicals.

2. Replace Gradually: Transition one product at a time to avoid overwhelming your skin with changes. Start with items like facial cleansers and moisturizers.

3. Opt for Gentle Cleansers: Look for sulfate-free options with nourishing ingredients like oatmeal or calendula.

4. Moisturize Naturally: Choose products with hydrating oils like jojoba or shea butter, which protect the skin without clogging pores.

5. DIY Solutions: Make your own skincare with simple ingredients like honey, yogurt, and essential oils.

Detoxifying Your Household Products

Skin health is influenced not just by what we apply topically but also by the environment we live in. Cleaning products, air fresheners, and laundry detergents often release allergens and irritants that impact skin conditions.

Switch to Natural Cleaners: Replace chemical-based cleaners with vinegar, baking soda, and lemon juice.

Eliminate Synthetic Air Fresheners: Use essential oil diffusers or natural potpourri.

Opt for Plant-Based Detergents: These are gentler on fabrics and skin.

Creating a Long-Term Healthy Environment

Consistency is key when transitioning to natural products. By reducing your overall exposure to toxins, you'll create a supportive environment for your skin to heal. Combine this approach with a healthy diet, stress management, and hydration to maximize results.

Switching to natural skincare and household products is an empowering step in managing seborrheic dermatitis. It not only reduces irritants but also aligns with a holistic approach to health and wellness. Start small, stay committed, and enjoy the benefits of a toxin-free lifestyle.

6.3 Creating a Skin-Healthy Living Space

Your living environment plays a critical role in the health of your skin, especially when dealing with conditions like seborrheic dermatitis.

Harmful chemicals, allergens, and irritants in your home can aggravate sensitive skin and hinder healing. Detoxifying your living space is a powerful step toward supporting your body's natural ability to heal and maintain healthy skin. **Below is a guide to creating a skin-friendly environment that promotes healing and prevents flare-ups.**

1. Switch to Natural Cleaning Products

Harsh cleaning agents often contain irritants such as synthetic fragrances, sulfates, and strong chemicals that can worsen skin inflammation.

Opt for natural alternatives: Use products with simple, plant-based ingredients like white vinegar, baking soda, and essential oils for cleaning.

Avoid synthetic fragrances: Choose unscented or naturally scented products to reduce exposure to skin-irritating chemicals.

Make your own cleaners: Mix vinegar and water for an all-purpose cleaner or baking soda with water for scrubbing.

2. Improve Air Quality

Airborne irritants like dust, mold, and chemicals can negatively impact your skin.

Ventilation: Keep windows open whenever possible to let in fresh air. Use exhaust fans in bathrooms and kitchens to reduce humidity and prevent mold growth.

Air purifiers: Invest in an air purifier with a HEPA filter to trap dust, pet dander, and other allergens.

Houseplants: Certain plants, such as spider plants and peace lilies, naturally filter toxins from the air.

3. Choose Skin-Safe Fabrics and Furniture

Materials that come into contact with your skin can irritate or soothe, depending on their quality.

Use organic fabrics: Opt for bedding, towels, and clothing made from organic cotton, bamboo, or linen, as these are free of harsh dyes and chemicals.

Avoid synthetic materials: Polyester and other synthetic fibers may trap sweat and irritate sensitive skin.

Natural furniture: Select furniture made from untreated or minimally treated wood to avoid chemical exposure.

4. Eliminate Toxic Personal Care Products

Many conventional personal care products are loaded with fragrances, alcohol, and preservatives that can disrupt the skin's natural barrier.

Read labels carefully: Avoid products with parabens, sulfates, phthalates, and synthetic dyes.

Simplify skincare routines: Stick to a gentle, natural cleanser and a moisturizer made with ingredients like aloe vera or shea butter.

Homemade alternatives: Create your own skincare products using simple, safe ingredients like coconut oil or oatmeal.

5. Control Humidity Levels

Both excessive dryness and high humidity can trigger seborrheic dermatitis flare-ups.

Use a humidifier: In dry climates or during winter, a humidifier helps maintain skin-friendly moisture levels in the air.

Dehumidify damp spaces: In humid areas, dehumidifiers can reduce excess moisture and prevent mold, a common irritant.

6. Reduce Exposure to Allergens

Allergens like dust mites, pet dander, and mold can exacerbate skin inflammation.

Regular cleaning: Vacuum and dust weekly, and wash bedding frequently in hot water.

Hypoallergenic bedding: Invest in hypoallergenic mattress covers and pillowcases.

Mold control: Address leaks and moisture issues promptly to prevent mold growth in your home.

7. Practice Minimalism

Clutter traps dust and allergens, making it harder to maintain a clean, skin-friendly environment.

Declutter regularly: Remove unnecessary items that collect dust or are hard to clean.

Opt for easy-to-clean surfaces: Choose furniture and flooring materials that are smooth and washable, like hardwood or tile.

8. Create a Calm and Stress-Free Space

Stress is a common trigger for seborrheic dermatitis, and your living space should help you relax.

Natural lighting: Maximize natural light to create a soothing environment.

Comfortable design: Include soft, calming colors and comfortable furniture to promote relaxation.

Mindful spaces: Dedicate areas for mindfulness practices, such as meditation or yoga, to help reduce stress.

Detoxifying your living space is an essential part of a holistic approach to managing and preventing seborrheic dermatitis. By creating a clean, natural, and soothing environment, you support your skin's healing process and reduce the risk of flare-ups. Small changes in your home can make a big difference in achieving lasting skin health.

Chapter 7

Building a Flare-Free Skincare Routine

7.1 Daily Skincare Practices for Seborrheic Dermatitis

Seborrheic dermatitis can be challenging to manage, but a consistent, thoughtful skincare routine can significantly reduce flares and support healing. This guide provides practical steps to build a gentle, effective daily routine tailored to soothe and protect sensitive skin.

1. Morning Routine

Start your day with a clean and calm foundation.

Cleanse Gently:
Use a mild, sulfate-free cleanser designed for sensitive skin. Look for ingredients like aloe vera or calendula, which soothe irritation. Avoid harsh soaps or cleansers with alcohol, as they can strip the skin of natural oils.

Tip: Wash with lukewarm water—hot water can worsen dryness and inflammation.

Moisturize Wisely:
Apply a lightweight, non-comedogenic moisturizer immediately after cleansing to lock in hydration. Choose one containing ceramides or hyaluronic acid to restore the skin barrier.

Protect with Sunscreen:
Even on cloudy days, apply a mineral-based sunscreen (like zinc oxide or titanium dioxide). Sun damage can worsen flares and irritate the skin.

2. Evening Routine

At night, your skin regenerates. A calming routine can enhance this process.

Cleanse Again:

Remove dirt, oil, and environmental pollutants accumulated during the day. Stick to the same gentle cleanser from your morning routine.

Targeted Care:
If recommended by your healthcare provider, apply medicated treatments such as an antifungal cream or hydrocortisone for active flares. Always use these sparingly and under supervision to avoid overuse.

Deep Moisturization:
Opt for a slightly richer moisturizer at night to provide deep hydration. Natural options like shea butter or jojoba oil are excellent for soothing dry, flaky patches.

3. Weekly or Biweekly Practices

Incorporate these steps to address specific concerns and maintain balance.

Exfoliate Mildly:

Use a gentle, chemical exfoliant like lactic acid or salicylic acid once a week to remove dead skin and reduce flaking. Avoid physical scrubs—they can irritate sensitive areas.

Hydrating Masks:
Apply a soothing, hydrating mask with ingredients like oat extract or honey to replenish and calm the skin.

4. Lifestyle Enhancements

Good skincare goes beyond what you apply to your face.

Stay Hydrated:
Drink plenty of water to keep your skin hydrated from within.

Manage Stress:
Stress can trigger seborrheic dermatitis. Practice relaxation techniques like meditation or yoga to stay calm.

Eat a Balanced Diet:
Incorporate anti-inflammatory foods like leafy greens, omega-3-rich fish, and probiotics. Avoid excessive sugar or processed foods, which can worsen inflammation.

5. Choosing Skincare Products

Select products that are free of fragrances, dyes, and irritants. **Look for labels such as:**

"Hypoallergenic"

"Dermatologist-tested"

"Suitable for sensitive skin"

6. Monitor and Adjust

Everyone's skin is unique. Keep a skincare journal to track your routine, products, and triggers. This will help you identify what works and make adjustments as needed.

A daily skincare routine for seborrheic dermatitis doesn't have to be complicated. Focus on gentle cleansing, consistent moisturization, and sun protection. Combined with a healthy lifestyle and mindful product choices, these practices can promote healing and prevent flares, allowing your skin to thrive naturally.

7.2 How to Properly Cleanse, Moisturize, and Protect

Seborrheic dermatitis can be a frustrating condition, but a thoughtful, natural skincare routine can significantly reduce flare-ups and discomfort. By focusing on gentle cleansing, effective moisturizing, and daily protection, you can support your skin's health and prevent irritation. **Here's a step-by-step guide:**

Step 1: Cleanse Gently

Cleansing is the foundation of any skincare routine. For those with seborrheic dermatitis, it's critical to avoid harsh soaps and cleansers that can strip the skin of its natural oils and cause irritation.

1. Choose the Right Cleanser:
Look for a mild, sulfate-free, pH-balanced cleanser. Ingredients such as aloe vera, chamomile, or calendula can soothe inflammation. For natural remedies, consider using raw honey as a gentle antibacterial cleanser or diluted apple cider vinegar as a rinse to restore the skin's natural pH.

2. Avoid Hot Water:
Use lukewarm water when washing your face or affected areas. Hot water can dry out the skin and exacerbate symptoms.

3. Be Gentle:
Massage the cleanser onto the skin with your fingertips using circular motions. Avoid scrubbing or using abrasive tools that can irritate sensitive areas.

4. Rinse Thoroughly:

Ensure no residue is left behind, as this can trigger flare-ups. Pat your skin dry with a soft, clean towel—do not rub.

Step 2: Moisturize Effectively

Moisturizing helps restore the skin barrier, keeping your skin hydrated and reducing flaking and irritation. The right moisturizer will lock in moisture without clogging pores or triggering breakouts.

1. Select a Natural Moisturizer:
Opt for products free of synthetic fragrances, dyes, and alcohol. Ingredients like shea butter, coconut oil, jojoba oil, or squalane are excellent natural moisturizers that soothe and hydrate the skin.

2. Apply While Skin is Damp:
Immediately after cleansing, apply a thin layer of moisturizer to slightly damp skin. This helps seal in moisture and enhances absorption.

3. Address Specific Areas:

If certain areas are more prone to flaking or redness, give them extra attention. For persistent patches, a small amount of pure aloe vera gel can provide relief and promote healing.

4. Test New Products:

Always do a patch test before introducing a new moisturizer to your routine to ensure it won't irritate your skin.

Step 3: Protect Your Skin Daily

Protecting your skin from environmental factors is essential to minimize flare-ups. Sun exposure, pollution, and even harsh weather can worsen seborrheic dermatitis symptoms.

1. Use a Mineral Sunscreen:

Choose a non-comedogenic sunscreen with zinc oxide or titanium dioxide. These physical blockers are gentle and less likely to cause irritation than chemical sunscreens.

2. Avoid Harsh Chemicals:
Steer clear of skincare and household products containing synthetic fragrances, parabens, and sulfates. These can disrupt your skin's natural barrier and increase sensitivity.

3. Hydrate Inside and Out:
Drink plenty of water throughout the day to keep your skin hydrated. Use a humidifier in dry climates to maintain moisture in the air and prevent skin dehydration.

4. Protect Against Harsh Weather:
In cold or windy conditions, cover your skin with soft, breathable fabrics to prevent irritation. Apply a thicker layer of moisturizer as a barrier before stepping outside.

Additional Tips for Long-Term Management

Stick to a Routine: Consistency is key. Follow your cleansing, moisturizing, and protecting steps daily, even if your skin is clear.

Monitor Triggers: Keep track of foods, stressors, or environmental factors that may cause flare-ups, and avoid them when possible.

Choose Gentle Exfoliation: If necessary, use a mild, natural exfoliant (such as oatmeal or a soft washcloth) once a week to remove dead skin cells without aggravating your condition.

Incorporate Antifungal Support: Since seborrheic dermatitis may be linked to an overgrowth of yeast, consider products with tea tree oil or natural antifungal properties. Always dilute tea tree oil before use to avoid irritation.

By focusing on these simple yet effective steps, you can build a skincare routine that supports your skin's natural healing process, reduces flare-ups, and promotes lasting health.

7.3 Adjusting Your Routine During Flare-Ups
Seborrheic dermatitis can present unique challenges, especially during flare-ups when symptoms like redness, irritation, and flaking

intensify. Adjusting your skincare routine during these times is crucial for soothing discomfort and preventing worsening symptoms. **Here's a step-by-step guide to help you build an effective, flare-free skincare routine:**

1. Prioritize Gentle Cleansing

During a flare-up, avoid harsh soaps or cleansers that strip the skin of natural oils. **Opt for:**

Mild, pH-balanced cleansers: Look for sulfate-free and fragrance-free options. Ingredients like aloe vera or chamomile can help calm irritation.

Warm, not hot water: Use lukewarm water to cleanse, as hot water can exacerbate dryness and inflammation.

Tip: Cleanse twice daily—once in the morning and once before bed—to remove buildup without over-drying.

2. Moisturize Consistently

Hydration is key to protecting the skin barrier and reducing flaking. Use a lightweight, non-comedogenic moisturizer that contains:

Ceramides: To restore the skin barrier.

Hyaluronic acid: For deep hydration.

Colloidal oatmeal: To reduce itching and inflammation.

Apply moisturizer immediately after cleansing while the skin is still slightly damp to lock in moisture.

3. Target Flare-Ups with Spot Treatments

Focus on calming active inflammation by incorporating gentle treatments such as:

Natural antifungals: Tea tree oil diluted in a carrier oil (like jojoba or sweet almond oil) may help address the underlying yeast imbalance.

Soothing agents: Apply calendula cream or aloe vera gel to calm redness and irritation.

Note: Always do a patch test before using new products to avoid further irritation.

4. Avoid Known Triggers

Certain ingredients or habits can worsen symptoms during a flare-up. **Steer clear of:**

- Alcohol-based toners or astringents.

- Synthetic fragrances and dyes.

- Over-exfoliation, which can irritate already-sensitive skin.

Instead, simplify your routine and stick to products with minimal, skin-friendly ingredients.

5. Protect Your Skin

Environmental factors like wind, cold weather, or sun exposure can aggravate flare-ups. **Protect your skin by:**

Using sunscreen: Choose a mineral-based sunscreen (zinc oxide or titanium dioxide) that's gentle on sensitive skin.

Wearing a hat or scarf: To shield the face during harsh weather conditions.

6. Incorporate Proactive Care

While treating flare-ups, include habits that can minimize recurrence:

Scalp care: If seborrheic dermatitis affects your scalp, use a mild anti-dandruff shampoo with natural ingredients like tea tree oil or salicylic acid.

Balanced diet: Include foods rich in omega-3 fatty acids, zinc, and antioxidants to support skin health from the inside out.

Stress management: Practice mindfulness or relaxation techniques to reduce stress, which is a common trigger.

7. Stay Consistent but Flexible

Building a flare-free skincare routine is about consistency, but you must also be adaptable to your skin's changing needs. If a product or method causes irritation, stop immediately and return to the basics: gentle cleansing, hydration, and protection.

Flare-ups are a normal part of living with seborrheic dermatitis, but they don't have to derail your skincare goals. By focusing on gentle, natural, and effective solutions, you can manage symptoms and support your skin's healing process. Adjust your routine thoughtfully, listen to your skin, and embrace a holistic approach to long-term relief.

Chapter 8

Healing From Within: Supplements and Nutritional Support

8.1 Key Vitamins and Minerals for Skin Health

Seborrheic dermatitis is a skin condition that often reflects deeper imbalances in the body, including nutrient deficiencies. Nourishing your skin from the inside out with key vitamins and minerals can play a significant role in healing and prevention. **Here's a comprehensive guide to essential nutrients and how they support skin health.**

1. Vitamin D: The Sunshine Vitamin

Vitamin D supports the immune system and helps regulate inflammation, both of which are crucial in managing seborrheic dermatitis.

How It Helps: It reduces skin redness and flakiness by promoting skin barrier function and calming inflammation.

Sources:

- Sunlight exposure (15–20 minutes daily)

- Fatty fish like salmon and mackerel

- Fortified foods like milk and cereals

- Supplements, especially during winter or if you have limited sun exposure

2. Vitamin E: The Skin Protector

Vitamin E is a powerful antioxidant that helps repair skin damage and protect against free radicals.

How It Helps: It soothes irritated skin and promotes healing of dry, flaky patches.

Sources:

- Nuts and seeds (almonds, sunflower seeds)
- Vegetable oils (olive oil, sunflower oil)
- Leafy greens like spinach and kale
- Supplements for targeted skin support

3. Biotin (Vitamin B7): The Skin, Hair, and Nail Booster

Biotin is vital for maintaining healthy skin by supporting cell renewal.

How It Helps: Prevents dryness, cracking, and flakiness often associated with seborrheic dermatitis.

Sources:

- Eggs (especially yolks)

- Nuts and seeds

- Sweet potatoes

- Biotin-rich supplements if deficiency is suspected

4. Zinc: The Skin Healer

Zinc plays a key role in wound healing, reducing inflammation, and controlling oil production.

How It Helps: It helps balance sebum production and fights fungal overgrowth, a common trigger for seborrheic dermatitis.

Sources:

- Shellfish (oysters, crab)

- Pumpkin seeds

- Meat (beef, chicken)

- Zinc supplements if dietary intake is inadequate

5. Selenium: The Antioxidant Mineral

Selenium helps protect skin cells from oxidative damage and supports a healthy scalp.

How It Helps: It reduces inflammation and works with other antioxidants like Vitamin E to combat skin issues.

Sources:

- Brazil nuts (just 1–2 nuts daily can meet your needs)

- Tuna and sardines

- Eggs

- Supplements, especially if deficiencies are diagnosed

6. Omega-3 Fatty Acids: The Inflammation Fighters

Omega-3s are essential fatty acids that help reduce inflammation and promote skin hydration.

How It Helps: They soothe redness and irritation while improving overall skin elasticity.

Sources:

- Fatty fish (salmon, sardines)

- Flaxseeds and chia seeds

- Walnuts

- Fish oil or algae-based supplements

7. Vitamin A: The Skin Repair Vitamin

Vitamin A supports skin regeneration and maintains the integrity of the skin barrier.

How It Helps: It reduces flakiness and supports the repair of damaged skin cells.

Sources:

- Sweet potatoes, carrots, and pumpkins (beta-carotene)

- Liver and eggs

- Dark leafy greens

- Supplements (preferably as beta-carotene to avoid toxicity)

8. Probiotics: The Gut-Skin Connection

Healthy gut flora plays a significant role in skin health by managing inflammation and supporting immunity.

How It Helps: Probiotics improve digestion and nutrient absorption, reducing skin flare-ups linked to seborrheic dermatitis.

Sources:

- Foods that undergo fermentation include items like yogurt, kefir, sauerkraut, and kimchi.

- Probiotic supplements tailored to skin health

9. Iron: The Oxygen Carrier

Iron is essential for delivering oxygen to skin cells, promoting healthy skin turnover.

How It Helps: Prevents skin dryness and paleness, often aggravated by seborrheic dermatitis.

Sources:

- Red meat and poultry

- Lentils and beans

- Spinach (combine with Vitamin C for better absorption)

- Iron supplements, if levels are low

10. Vitamin C: The Collagen Builder

Vitamin C enhances collagen production and protects skin from oxidative stress.

How It Helps: It boosts skin resilience and promotes faster healing of irritated areas.

Sources:

- Citrus fruits (oranges, lemons)

- Bell peppers

- Berries (strawberries, blueberries)

- Supplements for targeted antioxidant support

Tips for Optimal Nutrient Absorption

Pair fat-soluble vitamins (A, D, E, K) with healthy fats for better absorption.

Take probiotics alongside prebiotic-rich foods like bananas and onions for a synergistic effect.

Stay hydrated to support nutrient transport and skin hydration.

Consult a Professional

While dietary changes and supplements can help, it's essential to consult a healthcare provider to assess your unique needs. A blood test can identify deficiencies, ensuring that your approach to healing is both safe and effective.

By focusing on these vitamins and minerals, you can support your body's natural healing processes, improve skin health, and reduce the severity of seborrheic dermatitis. Healing truly starts from within.

8.2 Probiotics and Gut Support

Seborrheic dermatitis has a strong connection to gut health. Many experts now recognize the gut as the cornerstone of overall wellness, including skin health. By nurturing the gut with probiotics and nutrient-rich foods, you can support the body's natural defenses, reduce inflammation, and promote healing from within.

The Gut-Skin Axis: How the Gut Affects Your Skin

The gut-skin axis refers to the direct link between gut health and skin conditions. Imbalances in gut bacteria, known as dysbiosis, can trigger inflammation throughout the body, including the skin. This imbalance may contribute to skin issues like seborrheic dermatitis. Strengthening the gut with probiotics and proper nutrition restores balance, reduces inflammation, and boosts the immune system, all of which are critical for healing and preventing flare-ups.

Probiotic Supplements: A Key to Balancing Gut Health

Probiotics are beneficial bacteria that help restore the natural balance of the gut microbiome. They improve digestion, enhance nutrient absorption, and support immune function—all of which influence skin health.

Top Probiotic Strains for Skin Health

When choosing a probiotic supplement, look for these strains that are specifically beneficial for skin conditions:

1. Lactobacillus rhamnosus: Helps reduce inflammation and strengthen the skin barrier.

2. Lactobacillus plantarum: Known for its ability to soothe skin irritation and support gut balance.

3. Bifidobacterium breve: Aids in reducing inflammation and boosting skin hydration.

4. Saccharomyces boulardii: A probiotic yeast that combats harmful gut bacteria and reduces skin flare-ups.

Tips for Choosing Probiotic Supplements

Look for a product with multiple strains and a high CFU (colony-forming units) count.

Choose probiotics with added prebiotics, like inulin or chicory root, to feed the beneficial bacteria.

Opt for trusted brands with transparent ingredient sourcing and testing

A Holistic Approach to Skin Healing

While probiotics and nutrition form the foundation of gut and skin health, the most effective approach combines these strategies with other natural skincare practices. By addressing the root causes of seborrheic dermatitis, you can support your body in achieving long-lasting healing and vibrant, clear skin.

Take the time to nourish your body from within, and your skin will reflect the health and balance you've cultivated.

8.3 The Role of Omega-3s and Antioxidants

Seborrheic dermatitis is a persistent skin condition that thrives on inflammation and oxidative stress within the body. While topical treatments address symptoms on the surface, true healing starts from within. Incorporating omega-3 fatty acids and antioxidants into your diet or supplement regimen can play a vital role in reducing inflammation, strengthening the skin barrier, and supporting long-term skin health.

Why Omega-3 Fatty Acids Matter

Omega-3 fatty acids, primarily found in fish oil, flaxseeds, and walnuts, are essential fats that our bodies cannot produce on their own. These fatty acids are known for their anti-inflammatory properties, making them a powerful ally in calming seborrheic dermatitis.

Reducing Inflammation: Chronic inflammation is a significant contributor to seborrheic dermatitis. Omega-3s reduce the production of inflammatory compounds in the body, helping to soothe irritated skin and minimize redness and flaking.

Improving Skin Barrier Function: A healthy skin barrier retains moisture and protects against external irritants. Omega-3s strengthen the skin's lipid layer, preventing dryness and reducing flare-ups.

Balancing Oil Production: Seborrheic dermatitis often thrives in oily areas of the skin. Omega-3s help regulate sebum production, creating a less favorable environment for yeast overgrowth, a common trigger for the condition.

Antioxidants: Protecting Against Oxidative Stress

Antioxidants are compounds that neutralize free radicals—unstable molecules that damage cells and accelerate inflammation. Seborrheic dermatitis sufferers often experience heightened oxidative stress, which weakens the skin and exacerbates symptoms.

Vitamin E: Found in nuts, seeds, and green leafy vegetables, vitamin E supports skin repair and reduces oxidative damage. It also works as a natural moisturizer, promoting smoother, healthier skin.

Vitamin C: This potent antioxidant, abundant in citrus fruits, berries, and bell peppers, boosts collagen production and strengthens skin resilience. It also supports immune function, helping the body fight off triggers like yeast overgrowth.

Selenium and Zinc: These trace minerals, found in foods like Brazil nuts and pumpkin seeds, are powerful antioxidants that reduce inflammation and support skin repair. Selenium also plays a role in regulating the skin's natural oil balance.

Polyphenols: Present in green tea, dark chocolate, and brightly colored fruits, polyphenols fight inflammation and protect skin cells from free radical damage.

How to Incorporate Omega-3s and Antioxidants

1. Dietary Sources:

Add fatty fish like salmon, mackerel, or sardines to your meals at least twice a week. For plant-based options, include chia seeds, flaxseeds, and walnuts.

Incorporate colorful fruits and vegetables into your daily diet to ensure a broad spectrum of antioxidants. Think berries, spinach, sweet potatoes, and broccoli.

Include nuts and seeds for their vitamin E, selenium, and healthy fats.

2. Supplements:

Fish Oil or Algal Oil Capsules: If dietary intake is insufficient, supplements can provide a concentrated source of omega-3s. Look for high-quality options with EPA and DHA.

Vitamin C and E Capsules: Choose supplements made from natural sources to complement your diet.

Zinc and Selenium: A balanced multivitamin or specific mineral supplement can ensure adequate intake.

3. Lifestyle Practices:

Avoid foods high in processed sugars and trans fats, which promote inflammation and oxidative stress.

Stay hydrated to support skin cell turnover and maintain elasticity.

Pair antioxidant-rich foods with healthy fats to enhance nutrient absorption (e.g., drizzle olive oil on a salad).

The Synergy of Omega-3s and Antioxidants

Omega-3s and antioxidants work hand-in-hand to create an internal environment conducive to healing. While omega-3s target inflammation at its root, antioxidants neutralize the oxidative stress that aggravates seborrheic dermatitis. Together, they not only alleviate symptoms but also promote overall skin health, reducing the likelihood of future flare-ups.

Healing from seborrheic dermatitis involves addressing the underlying causes of inflammation and oxidative stress. By incorporating omega-3 fatty acids and antioxidants into your diet and supplement routine, you can support your body's natural healing processes and achieve healthier, clearer skin. This approach complements topical treatments, creating a balanced and sustainable path to skin wellness.

Chapter 9

Preventing Future Flare-Ups

Seborrheic dermatitis thrives when your skin and body are out of balance. Preventing future flare-ups requires consistent care and mindfulness of the factors that can worsen the condition. Developing a tailored routine of skincare, diet, and stress management will help keep your skin healthy and resilient. Regularly moisturize your skin using gentle, natural products, avoid harsh chemicals, and protect your skin from extreme weather conditions. Consistency in your care routine is essential.

Identifying and Avoiding Triggers

The key to long-term management lies in recognizing and avoiding personal triggers. **Common triggers include:**

Environmental Factors: Cold, dry air or high humidity can worsen symptoms.

Stress and Fatigue: Mental and physical stress can disrupt your skin's natural barrier, leading to flare-ups.

Dietary Sensitivities: Certain foods, especially those high in sugar, processed fats, or alcohol, can provoke inflammation.

Skincare Products: Harsh soaps, fragrances, and synthetic chemicals can irritate the skin.

Keep a journal to track what you eat, your environment, and your symptoms. This will help you identify patterns and make necessary adjustments to your lifestyle.

Maintaining a Balanced Diet and Lifestyle

Your diet and overall lifestyle play a vital role in preventing seborrheic dermatitis. **Focus on these essentials:**

1. Anti-Inflammatory Foods: Incorporate foods rich in omega-3 fatty acids, such as salmon, flaxseeds, and walnuts, which support healthy skin.

2. Gut Health: A strong connection exists between gut health and skin health. Consume probiotics through fermented foods like yogurt, kefir, and sauerkraut to maintain a balanced gut microbiome.

3. Stay hydrated by consuming ample water to ensure your skin remains moisturized from the inside out.

4. Stress Management: Incorporate mindfulness practices like meditation, yoga, or deep breathing to reduce stress levels.

5. Regular Exercise: Engage in moderate physical activity to boost circulation and support overall skin health.

Long-Term Strategies for Healthy, Flare-Free Skin

Long-term management requires a holistic approach. Implement these strategies to ensure **lasting results:**

Commit to a Simple, Natural Skincare Routine: Use mild, sulfate-free cleansers and nourish your skin with natural oils like coconut or jojoba. Avoid over-washing, which can strip your skin of natural oils.

Periodic Detoxification: Evaluate your environment for potential irritants, such as household cleaning products or laundry detergents. Replace them with natural, non-toxic alternatives.

Seasonal Adjustments: Adapt your skincare and hydration routines to align with seasonal changes. For instance, use heavier moisturizers in winter and lighter ones in summer.

Skin-Friendly Habits: Avoid scratching or picking at affected areas to prevent infection or scarring.

Professional Guidance: Consult a dermatologist or holistic practitioner for guidance tailored to your unique skin needs.

By integrating these practices into your daily life, you can support healthy skin, reduce flare-ups, and enjoy long-term relief from seborrheic dermatitis. Thoughtful prevention and a proactive approach are the keys to lasting results.

Printed in Dunstable, United Kingdom